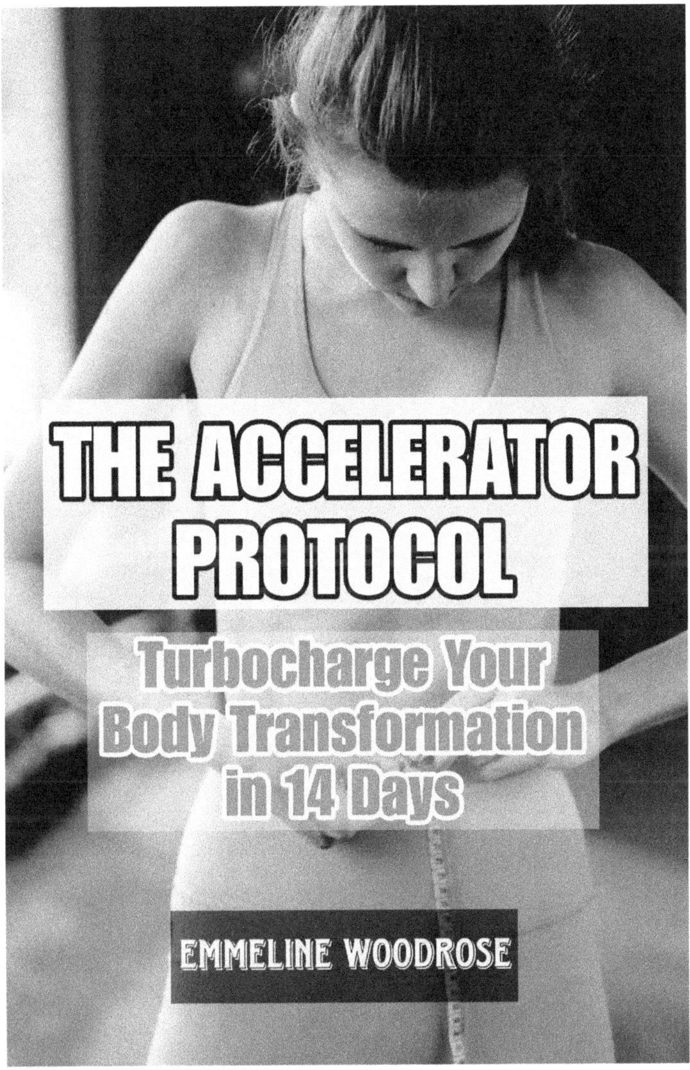

THE ACCELERATOR PROTOCOL

Turbocharge Your Body Transformation in 14 Days

EMMELINE WOODROSE

THE ACCELERATED LEANNESS PROTOCOL

Turbocharge Your Body Transformation in 14 Days

BY
EMMELINE WOODROSE

TABLE CONTENT

INTRODUCTION

Are you tired of trying fad diet after fad diet, only to see no results? Have you been struggling to lose those stubborn pounds and get the lean, toned physique you've always wanted? Look no further than the Accelerated Leanness Protocol, a revolutionary 14-day program designed to turbocharge your body transformation and help you achieve your dream body in record time.

An Inspiring Story of Transformation

Let me share with you the story of Sarah, a 35-year-old working mom who had all but given up on ever getting back her pre-baby body. Sarah had tried a ton of diets and workout plans, just like many of us, but nothing worked for her. She was constantly exhausted, carrying around an extra 25 pounds that just wouldn't budge.

That all changed when Sarah discovered The Accelerated Leanness Protocol. At first, she was skeptical—after all, how could a 14-day program deliver the kind of results she had been chasing for years? But with nothing to lose, she decided to give it a shot.

The first few days were tough, as Sarah's body adjusted to the unique combination of strategic nutrition, high-intensity workouts, and targeted supplementation that lie at the heart of The Accelerated Leanness Protocol. Visible changes in the mirror that she was already starting to see motivated her to stick with it.

By the end of the 14 days, Sarah had lost an incredible 12 pounds of stubborn fat while gaining lean muscle definition she hadn't seen since her early 20s. But even more importantly, she had regained her energy, her confidence, and her zest for life. The Accelerated Leanness Protocol had not only transformed her body but also her entire outlook on health and wellness.

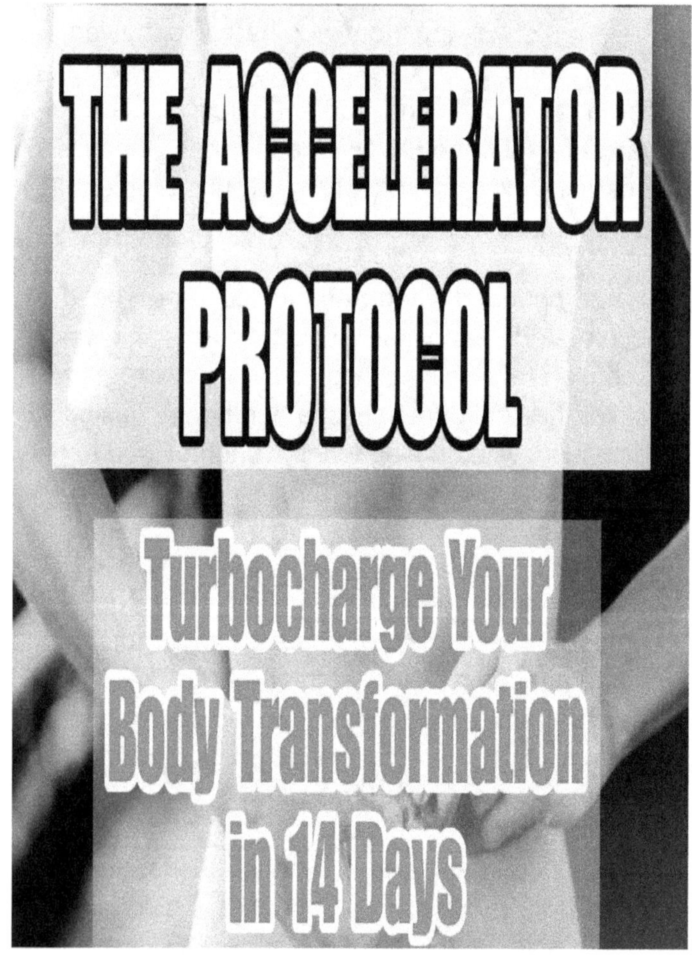

The Science Behind The Accelerated Leanness Protocol

So, what makes The Accelerated Leanness Protocol so effective? The secret lies in its multi-pronged approach, which tackles weight loss and body transformation from every angle.

Strategic Nutrition

At the core of The Accelerated Leanness Protocol is a carefully designed nutrition plan that optimizes your body's fat-burning potential. By strategically cycling periods of low-carb, high-fat eating with strategic carb refeeds, you'll prime your metabolism to burn fat for fuel while preserving precious muscle mass.

But this isn't just another ketogenic diet. The Accelerated Leanness Protocol takes things a step further by incorporating nutrient-dense, anti-inflammatory foods that help reduce bloating and combat the hormonal imbalances that often sabotage weight loss efforts.

High-Intensity Workouts

Nutrition is just one piece of the puzzle. To truly turbocharge your body's transformation, you need to pair it with the right kind of exercise. That's why The Accelerated Leanness Protocol includes a series of high-intensity workouts designed to shock your body into burning fat while building lean, metabolically active muscle.

These workouts are short, intense, and can be done anywhere with minimal equipment. But don't let their simplicity fool you; they'll push your body to its limits, igniting a powerful fat-burning furnace that will continue to smolder long after you've left the gym.

Targeted Supplementation

Finally, the Accelerated Leanness Protocol incorporates a strategic supplementation plan to support your body's natural fat-burning processes and accelerate your results. From thermogenic fat burners to cortisol-lowering adaptogens, these carefully selected supplements work synergistically with your nutrition and exercise plan to create an environment primed for maximum fat loss and muscle growth.

Why The Accelerated Leanness Protocol Works

But The Accelerated Leanness Protocol isn't just a collection of random diet and exercise tips; it's a carefully crafted system designed to overcome the specific physiological and psychological barriers that often sabotage our weight loss efforts.

Overcoming Metabolic Adaptation

One of the biggest challenges when it comes to losing weight is something called "metabolic adaptation." As you lose weight, your body adapts by slowing down your metabolism, making it increasingly difficult to continue shedding pounds. This is why so many people hit a frustrating plateau after initial weight loss success.

The Accelerated Leanness Protocol tackles this issue head-on by strategically cycling your calorie and macronutrient intake, keeping your metabolism guessing and preventing it from adapting to a lower caloric baseline.

Combating Hormonal Imbalances

Another major roadblock to sustainable weight loss is hormonal imbalance. When hormones like cortisol, insulin, and leptin are out of whack, it can lead to increased appetite, stubborn fat storage, and a host of other issues that make it highly challenging to lose weight and maintain it.

The Accelerated Leanness Protocol addresses this by incorporating specific foods, supplements, and lifestyle strategies designed to balance your hormones and create an internal environment conducive to fat loss and muscle growth.

Harnessing the Power of Mindset

But perhaps most importantly, The Accelerated Leanness Protocol recognizes that sustainable weight loss and body transformation are as much a mental game as it are a physical one. That's why the program includes a powerful mindset component, equipping you with the tools and strategies you need to stay motivated, overcome self-sabotage, and develop the unshakable belief in yourself that is essential for lasting success.

The Results You Can Expect

So, what kind of results can you expect from The Accelerated Leanness Protocol? While individual results may vary, many participants report losing anywhere from 10 to 15 pounds of stubborn fat in just 14 days while simultaneously gaining lean muscle definition and a renewed sense of energy and vitality.

But the benefits of The Accelerated Leanness Protocol extend far beyond just physical transformation. By addressing the underlying hormonal, metabolic, and psychological factors that often sabotage weight loss efforts, you'll be setting yourself up for long-term success and a sustainable lifestyle change that will keep you looking and feeling your best for years to come.

The 14-Day Accelerated Leanness Protocol Breakdown

So, what exactly does The Accelerated Leanness Protocol entail? Below is a daily summary of what to anticipate:

Days 1-3: The Priming Phase

The first three days of the Accelerated Leanness Protocol are all about priming your body for the intense fat-burning phase to come. During this time, you'll focus on eliminating inflammatory foods, stabilizing your blood sugar, and gently easing your body into a state of nutritional ketosis.

Your nutrition plan during this phase will consist of:

- Low-carb, high-fat meals featuring nutrient-dense proteins like grass-fed beef, wild-caught fish, and pasture-raised eggs
- An abundance of low-carb vegetables like leafy greens, cruciferous veggies, and colorful peppers
- Healthy fats from sources like avocados, nuts, seeds, and olive oil
- Moderate amounts of low-glycemic fruits like berries and citrus

Your workouts during this phase will be relatively low-intensity, focusing on mobility and flexibility and getting your body primed for the more intense training to come.

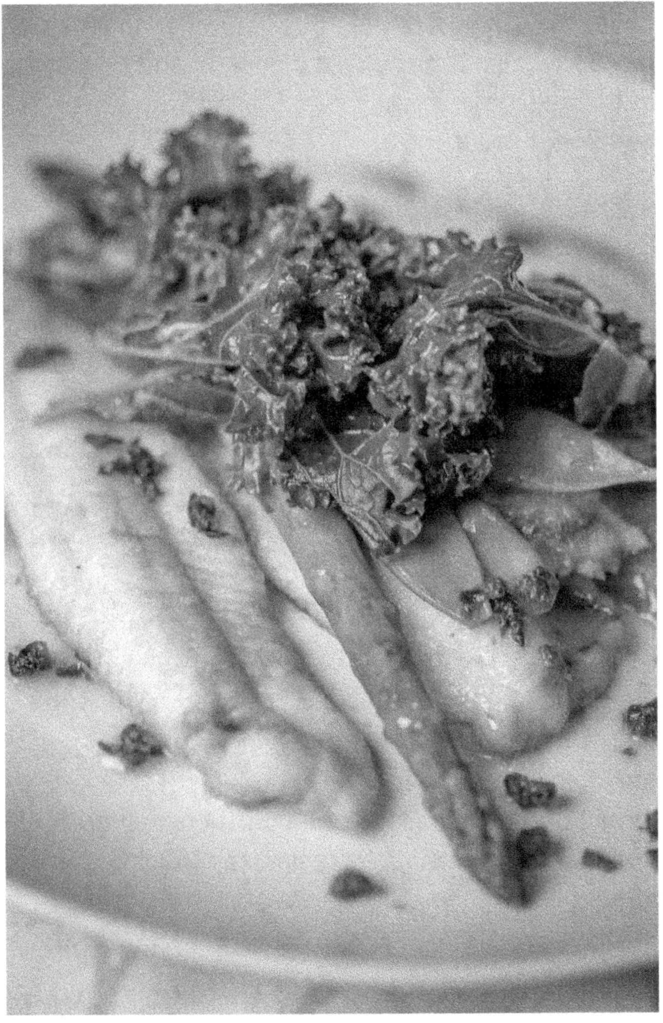

Days 4–10: The Fat-Burning Accelerator

This is where the real magic happens. During these seven days, you'll be pushing your body to its fat-burning limits through a combination of strategic nutrition, high-intensity workouts, and targeted supplementation.

Your nutrition plan during this phase will feature:

- The Accelerated Leanness Protocol will punctuate periods of your very low-carb intake with strategic carb refeeds to keep your metabolism revved through cyclical ketosis.
- An emphasis on nutrient-dense, anti-inflammatory foods like wild-caught seafood, leafy greens, and berries
- Thermogenic fat-burning supplements like green tea extract, cayenne pepper, and forskolin

Your workouts will be short, intense, and designed to maximize your body's fat-burning potential through techniques like high-intensity interval training (HIIT), metabolic resistance training, and strategically timed cardio sessions.

Days 11–14: The Peak Week

As you enter the final stretch of the Accelerated Leanness Protocol, it's time to really dial things in and push your body to its peak potential. During this "peak week," you'll be following a very specific nutrition and training plan designed to prime your body for maximum fat loss and reveal your hard-earned muscle definition.

Your nutrition plan during this phase will look something like this:

- A gradual increase in carbohydrate intake from clean sources like sweet potatoes, rice, and oats
- A continued emphasis on nutrient-dense proteins and healthy fats
- Strategic supplementation with muscle-sparing compounds like HMB and creatine

Your workouts will shift gears as well, with a greater focus on high-volume resistance training to really etch out those hard-earned muscle fibers. You'll also be incorporating specific depletion and dehydration protocols to achieve that coveted "peaked" look for your final physique reveal.

Success Stories and Testimonials

But don't just take my word for it. The Accelerated Leanness Protocol has already helped countless people, just like you, achieve incredible body transformations in record time.

A handful of their accounts are as follows:

Michael, 42

"I've been stuck in a rut for years, struggling to lose that stubborn belly fat no matter what I tried. The Accelerated Leanness Protocol was a game-changer for me. In just 14 days, I dropped 12 pounds and finally unveiled the six-pack abs I haven't seen since my 20s. But even better than the physical changes were the mental shifts—I feel more confident, energized, and in control of my health than ever before."

"As a busy mom of two, I thought getting my pre-baby body back was just a pipe dream. But The Accelerated Leanness Protocol proved me wrong. Not only did I lose 10 pounds of stubborn fat, but I also gained a newfound appreciation for how powerful our bodies can be when we give them the right tools and strategies. I've never felt better or more energized in my life!"

"I'll be honest, I was pretty skeptical about any program promising such dramatic results in just 14 days. But I decided to give The Accelerated Leanness Protocol a shot, and I'm so glad I did. Not only did I shed 14 pounds of unwanted fat, but I also gained a whole new perspective on healthy living that I know will stick with me for life."

Get Started Today

If you're ready to finally achieve the lean, toned, and confident body you've always wanted, it's time to take action and give The Accelerated Leanness Protocol a try. With its comprehensive, science-backed approach and proven track record of success, this 14-day program could very well be the last weight-loss solution you ever need.

But don't wait—the sooner you get started, the sooner you'll be on your way to a whole new you. Click the link below to purchase The Accelerated Leanness Protocol today and take the first step towards your ultimate body transformation!

Frequently Asked Questions

Is the Accelerated Leanness Protocol safe?

Absolutely! The Accelerated Leanness Protocol is designed with safety as a top priority. The Accelerated Leanness Protocol backs all of its nutrition, exercise, and supplementation protocols with science and bases them on proven, sustainable principles. However, as with any major lifestyle change, it's always a good idea to consult with your healthcare provider before getting started.

How much time will I need to commit?

One of the best things about the Accelerated Leanness Protocol is that it's designed to fit seamlessly into even the busiest of lifestyles. While you'll need to be diligent about following the nutrition plan and getting in your workouts, most people find that the program requires no more than 1-2 hours of dedicated time per day.

What kind of equipment do I need?

The Accelerated Leanness Protocol can be followed with minimal equipment; all you really need is a set of resistance bands, some space to move around, and access to a grocery store for your fresh, whole-food ingredients. Optional items like dumbbells or a pull-up bar can enhance your results, but they're not strictly necessary.

Is this program suitable for beginners?

Yes! The Accelerated Leanness Protocol is designed to be accessible and effective for people of all fitness levels. Whether you're a total newcomer to the world of health and fitness or a seasoned pro, the program will meet you where you're at and provide you with everything you need to succeed.

What kind of support is available?

When you purchase The Accelerated Leanness Protocol, you'll gain access to a private online community of like-minded individuals who are all on the same journey towards better health and fitness. In this community, you'll be able to connect with others, share your progress, ask questions, and receive ongoing support and motivation from certified coaches and fellow participants alike.

Take the First Step Today

If you're truly ready to transform your body and your life in just 14 days, the time to act is now. Don't let another day go by feeling frustrated, unhappy, and trapped in a body that doesn't reflect your true potential.

The Accelerated Leanness Protocol has already helped countless people, just like you, achieve incredible results in record time, and it can do the same for you. But you have to take that first, crucial step and commit to making a change.

So, what are you waiting for? Get your copy to get started on your ultimate body transformation journey today. Your leaner, more confident, and infinitely healthier self is just 14 days away!